Carbohydrate

Tracker

AF730775

Easy To Use

Food Journal

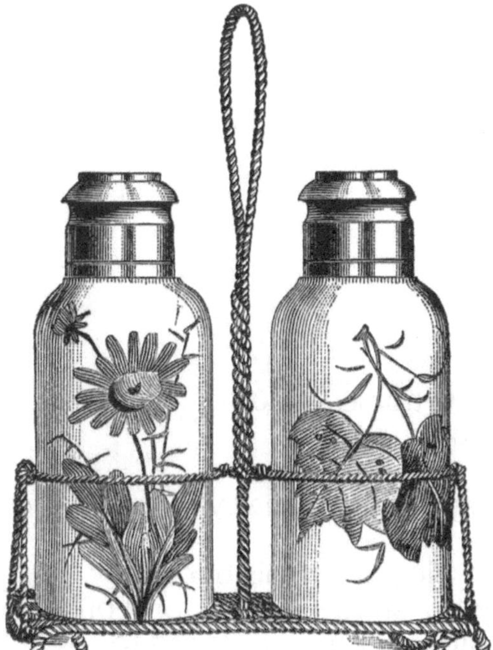

Diana Lynn

Published by D&D Graphics in 2017
First edition; First printing

ISBN: 978-0-9982413-2-6

Dedication

This is dedicated to everyone looking for an easy-to-use food journal.

Thank you, Evelyn, for being a great sister and for your support in the creation of this journal.

Thanks to my family, Don, Brian and Jeff, for putting up with me and the massive amount of time I spend on the computer creating. I love you all!

"Your diet is a bank account. Good food choices are good investments."

Bethenny Frankel

This book belongs to:

____

Start Date: ________________

Goals:

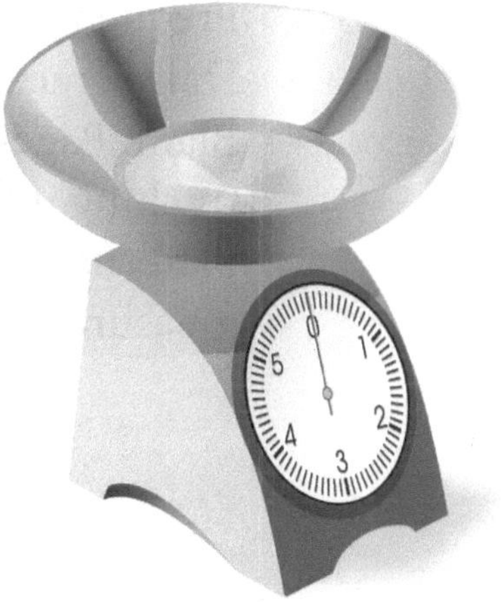

Weight: ______________

Carbs per day: _________

Water intake: __________

Steps per day: _________

Exercise minutes per day/week: __________

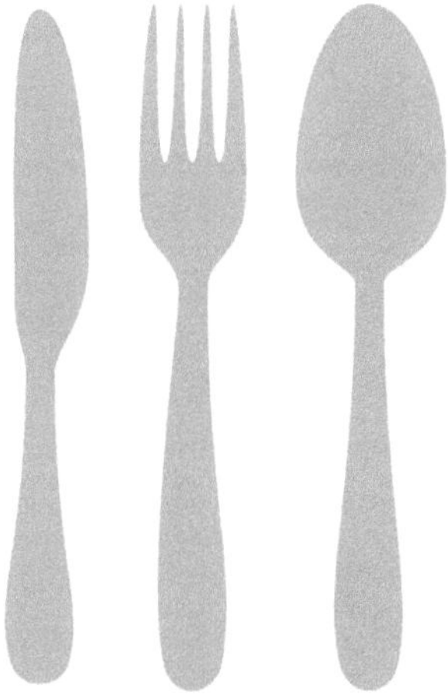

The Easy to Use Food Tracking Journal includes:

- Goal Sheet
- Sample pages
- Weight Tracking Logs
- Frequent Food List
- Daily Tracking Logs
- Blank Pages for notes, additional tracking information, noticeable patterns or habits, body measurements, recipes, quotes etc.

Tips:

1. Add up your carbs as you go. The running total will allow you to quickly calculate how many carbs you have left to consume before reaching your daily goal.
2. If you skip a day of food tracking, make a note at the top or bottom of the page as to why.
3. Circle the day of the week for quick reference.
4. Clipping the corner enables you to quickly locate your current page.
5. The daily tracking pages include spaces to log steps and exercise minutes.
6. Each glass represents eight ounces (or set your own measurement) of water. Mark the glasses as you drink, throughout the day.
7. Note the time you eat your meal or snack. This will show how often you eat. Do you eat at regular intervals or take too much time between meals? When you log your time you may notice patterns in your diet, such as overeating at dinner because you skipped lunch.
8. How do you feel today? Your mood can be an indicator of food choices. If you're rushed, it might explain the fish crackers. Or maybe you're tired? Sad because of bad news? Energized? Frustrated? By answering the question, you may find an eating pattern that you didn't know existed!
9. Add any other notes that may explain your day.

Sample Weight Tracking Log

Starting Weight: 200

Date	Current Weight	Loss/Gain	Overall Loss/Gain to date
Jan 3	199	-1	-1
Jan 10	194	-5	-6
Jan 14	195	+1	-5
Jan 21	190	-5	-10
Feb 5	196	-4	-14

Sample Frequent Food List

Amount	Food	Carbs
1 serv.	baked meatballs and green beans	7
1	breakfast burrito - peppers & onion	8

For quick reference, build a list of food items you frequently consume.

Sample Daily Tracking Log

Date: 5/12 M Tu W **(Th)** F Sa Su

Steps: 7,888 Exercise Minutes: 30

Water: 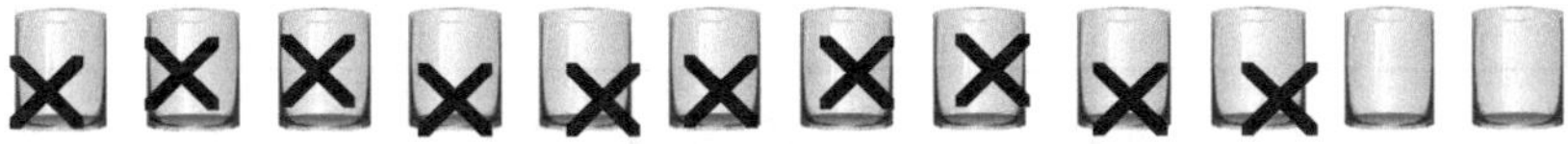

Time	Food Item	Carbs	Carbs Balance
7:15am	2 egg & sausage muffins	2	2
	Coffee with 1/2 & 1/2	1.3	3.3
10:10am	2 hard boiled egg	0	3.3
12:45pm	Broccoli salad	6.8	10.1
3:30pm	Beef Chili	8.2	18.3
5:50pm	Stuffed pepper	11	29.3
	2 oz. cheddar cheese	.8	30.1

How do you feel today? Frustrated! I seem to run into delays every where I turned.

Note: If used daily, there are enough tracking log sheets for approximately three months.

Weight Tracking Log

Starting Weight: ___________

Date	Current Weight	Loss/Gain	Overall Loss/Gain to date

Weight Tracking Log

Starting Weight: ___________

Date	Current Weight	Loss/Gain	Overall Loss/Gain to date

Frequent Food List

Amount	Food	Carbs

Frequent Food List

Amount	Food	Carbs

Daily Tracking Log Sheets

Date: __________ M Tu W Th F Sa Su

Steps: __________ Exercise Minutes: __________

Water:

Time	Food Item	Carbs	Carb Balance

How do you feel today?
(Notes)

Date: __________ M Tu W Th F Sa Su

clip corner here

Steps: __________ Exercise Minutes: __________

Water:

Time	Food Item	Carbs	Carb Balance

How do you feel today?

(Notes)

Date: __________ M Tu W Th F Sa Su

Steps: __________ Exercise Minutes: __________

Water:

Time	Food Item	Carbs	Carb Balance

How do you feel today?
(Notes)

Date: __________ M Tu W Th F Sa Su

clip corner here

Steps: __________ Exercise Minutes: __________

Water:

Time	Food Item	Carbs	Carb Balance

How do you feel today?

(Notes)

Date: __________ M Tu W Th F Sa Su

Steps: __________ Exercise Minutes: __________

Water:

Time	Food Item	Carbs	Carb Balance

How do you feel today?

(Notes)

Date: __________ M Tu W Th F Sa Su

clip corner here

Steps: __________ Exercise Minutes: __________

Water:

Time	Food Item	Carbs	Carb Balance

How do you feel today?

(Notes)

Date: __________ M Tu W Th F Sa Su

Steps: __________ Exercise Minutes: __________

Water:

Time	Food Item	Carbs	Carb Balance

How do you feel today?

(Notes)

Date: __________ M Tu W Th F Sa Su

clip corner here

Steps: __________ Exercise Minutes: __________

Water:

Time	Food Item	Carbs	Carb Balance

How do you feel today?

(Notes)

Date: ________ M Tu W Th F Sa Su

Steps: ________ Exercise Minutes: ________

Water:

Time	Food Item	Carbs	Carb Balance

How do you feel today?
(Notes)

clip corner here

Date: __________ M Tu W Th F Sa Su

Steps: __________ Exercise Minutes: __________

Water:

Time	Food Item	Carbs	Carb Balance

How do you feel today?

(Notes)

Date: __________ M Tu W Th F Sa Su

Steps: __________ Exercise Minutes: __________

Water: ☐ ☐ ☐ ☐ ☐ ☐ ☐ ☐ ☐ ☐ ☐ ☐

Time	Food Item	Carbs	Carb Balance

How do you feel today?

(Notes)

clip corner here

Date: __________ M Tu W Th F Sa Su

Steps: __________ Exercise Minutes: __________

Water:

Time	Food Item	Carbs	Carb Balance

How do you feel today?

(Notes)

Date: __________ M Tu W Th F Sa Su

Steps: __________ Exercise Minutes: __________

Water: ☐ ☐ ☐ ☐ ☐ ☐ ☐ ☐ ☐ ☐ ☐ ☐

Time	Food Item	Carbs	Carb Balance

How do you feel today?
(Notes)

Date: __________ M Tu W Th F Sa Su

clip corner here

Steps: __________ Exercise Minutes: __________

Water:

Time	Food Item	Carbs	Carb Balance

How do you feel today?

(Notes)

Date: __________ M Tu W Th F Sa Su

Steps: __________ Exercise Minutes: __________

Water:

Time	Food Item	Carbs	Carb Balance

How do you feel today?
(Notes)

clip corner here

Date: __________ M Tu W Th F Sa Su

Steps: __________ Exercise Minutes: __________

Water:

Time	Food Item	Carbs	Carb Balance

How do you feel today?

(Notes)

Date: __________ M Tu W Th F Sa Su

Steps: __________ Exercise Minutes: __________

Water:

Time	Food Item	Carbs	Carb Balance

How do you feel today?

(Notes)

Date: __________ M Tu W Th F Sa Su

clip corner here

Steps: __________ Exercise Minutes: __________

Water:

Time	Food Item	Carbs	Carb Balance

How do you feel today?

(Notes)

Date: __________ M Tu W Th F Sa Su

Steps: __________ Exercise Minutes: __________

Water:

Time	Food Item	Carbs	Carb Balance

How do you feel today?

(Notes)

Date: __________ M Tu W Th F Sa Su

clip corner here

Steps: __________ Exercise Minutes: __________

Water:

Time	Food Item	Carbs	Carb Balance

How do you feel today?

(Notes)

Date: __________ M Tu W Th F Sa Su

Steps: __________ Exercise Minutes: __________

Water:

Time	Food Item	Carbs	Carb Balance

How do you feel today?
(Notes)

Date: __________ M Tu W Th F Sa Su

clip corner here

Steps: __________ Exercise Minutes: __________

Water:

Time	Food Item	Carbs	Carb Balance

How do you feel today?

(Notes)

Date: __________ M Tu W Th F Sa Su

Steps: __________ Exercise Minutes: __________

Water:

Time	Food Item	Carbs	Carb Balance

How do you feel today?

(Notes)

clip corner here

Date: __________ M Tu W Th F Sa Su

Steps: __________ Exercise Minutes: __________

Water:

Time	Food Item	Carbs	Carb Balance

How do you feel today?

(Notes)

Date: __________ M Tu W Th F Sa Su

Steps: __________ Exercise Minutes: __________

Water:

Time	Food Item	Carbs	Carb Balance

How do you feel today?

(Notes)

Date: __________ M Tu W Th F Sa Su

clip corner here

Steps: __________ Exercise Minutes: __________

Water:

Time	Food Item	Carbs	Carb Balance

How do you feel today?

(Notes)

Date: __________ M Tu W Th F Sa Su

Steps: __________ Exercise Minutes: __________

Water:

Time	Food Item	Carbs	Carb Balance

How do you feel today?
(Notes)

Date: __________ M Tu W Th F Sa Su

clip corner here

Steps: __________ Exercise Minutes: __________

Water:

Time	Food Item	Carbs	Carb Balance

How do you feel today?

(Notes)

Date: __________ M Tu W Th F Sa Su

Steps: __________ Exercise Minutes: __________

Water:

Time	Food Item	Carbs	Carb Balance

How do you feel today?
(Notes)

Date: __________ M Tu W Th F Sa Su

clip corner here

Steps: __________ Exercise Minutes: __________

Water:

Time	Food Item	Carbs	Carb Balance

How do you feel today?

(Notes)

Date: __________ M Tu W Th F Sa Su

Steps: __________ Exercise Minutes: __________

Water:

Time	Food Item	Carbs	Carb Balance

How do you feel today?
(Notes)

Date: __________ M Tu W Th F Sa Su

clip corner here

Steps: __________ Exercise Minutes: __________

Water:

Time	Food Item	Carbs	Carb Balance

How do you feel today?

(Notes)

Date: __________ M Tu W Th F Sa Su

Steps: __________ Exercise Minutes: __________

Water:

Time	Food Item	Carbs	Carb Balance

How do you feel today?
(Notes)

Date: __________ M Tu W Th F Sa Su

clip corner here

Steps: __________ Exercise Minutes: __________

Water:

Time	Food Item	Carbs	Carb Balance

How do you feel today?

(Notes)

Date: __________ M Tu W Th F Sa Su

Steps: __________ Exercise Minutes: __________

Water: 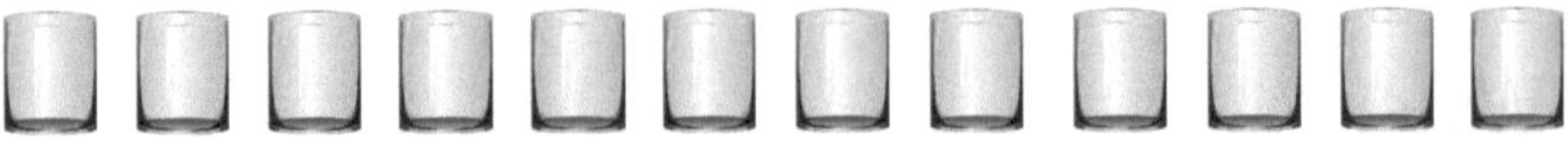

Time	Food Item	Carbs	Carb Balance

How do you feel today?

(Notes)

Date: __________ M Tu W Th F Sa Su

clip corner here

Steps: __________ Exercise Minutes: __________

Water:

Time	Food Item	Carbs	Carb Balance

How do you feel today?

(Notes)

Date: __________ M Tu W Th F Sa Su

Steps: __________ Exercise Minutes: __________

Water: 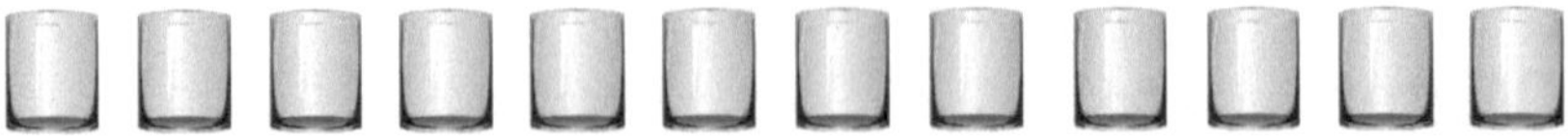

Time	Food Item	Carbs	Carb Balance

How do you feel today?

(Notes)

clip corner here

Date: __________ M Tu W Th F Sa Su

Steps: __________ Exercise Minutes: __________

Water:

Time	Food Item	Carbs	Carb Balance

How do you feel today?

(Notes)

Date: __________ M Tu W Th F Sa Su

Steps: __________ Exercise Minutes: __________

Water:

Time	Food Item	Carbs	Carb Balance

How do you feel today?

(Notes)

clip corner here

Date: __________ M Tu W Th F Sa Su

Steps: __________ Exercise Minutes: __________

Water:

Time	Food Item	Carbs	Carb Balance

How do you feel today?
(Notes)

Date: __________ M Tu W Th F Sa Su

Steps: __________ Exercise Minutes: __________

Water:

Time	Food Item	Carbs	Carb Balance

How do you feel today?

(Notes)

Date: __________ M Tu W Th F Sa Su

clip corner here

Steps: __________ Exercise Minutes: __________

Water:

Time	Food Item	Carbs	Carb Balance

How do you feel today?

(Notes)

Date: __________ M Tu W Th F Sa Su

Steps: __________ Exercise Minutes: __________

Water:

Time	Food Item	Carbs	Carb Balance

How do you feel today?
(Notes)

clip corner here

Date: __________ M Tu W Th F Sa Su

Steps: __________ Exercise Minutes: __________

Water:

Time	Food Item	Carbs	Carb Balance

How do you feel today?

(Notes)

Date: __________ M Tu W Th F Sa Su

Steps: __________ Exercise Minutes: __________

Water:

Time	Food Item	Carbs	Carb Balance

How do you feel today?

(Notes)

clip corner here

Date: __________ M Tu W Th F Sa Su

Steps: __________ Exercise Minutes: __________

Water:

Time	Food Item	Carbs	Carb Balance

How do you feel today?

(Notes)

Date: __________ M Tu W Th F Sa Su

Steps: __________ Exercise Minutes: __________

Water:

Time	Food Item	Carbs	Carb Balance

How do you feel today?

(Notes)

clip corner here

Date: __________ M Tu W Th F Sa Su

Steps: __________ Exercise Minutes: __________

Water:

Time	Food Item	Carbs	Carb Balance

How do you feel today?
(Notes)

Date: __________ M Tu W Th F Sa Su

Steps: __________ Exercise Minutes: __________

Water:

Time	Food Item	Carbs	Carb Balance

How do you feel today?

(Notes)

Date: __________ M Tu W Th F Sa Su

clip corner here

Steps: __________ Exercise Minutes: __________

Water:

Time	Food Item	Carbs	Carb Balance

How do you feel today?

(Notes)

Date: ________ M Tu W Th F Sa Su

Steps: ________ Exercise Minutes: ________

Water:

Time	Food Item	Carbs	Carb Balance

How do you feel today?

(Notes)

clip corner here

Date: __________ M Tu W Th F Sa Su

Steps: __________ Exercise Minutes: __________

Water:

Time	Food Item	Carbs	Carb Balance

How do you feel today?
(Notes)

Date: __________ M Tu W Th F Sa Su

Steps: __________ Exercise Minutes: __________

Water:

Time	Food Item	Carbs	Carb Balance

How do you feel today?
(Notes)

clip corner here

Date: __________ M Tu W Th F Sa Su

Steps: __________ Exercise Minutes: __________

Water:

Time	Food Item	Carbs	Carb Balance

How do you feel today?

(Notes)

Date: __________ M Tu W Th F Sa Su

Steps: __________ Exercise Minutes: __________

Water:

Time	Food Item	Carbs	Carb Balance

How do you feel today?

(Notes)

clip corner here

Date: __________ M Tu W Th F Sa Su

Steps: __________ Exercise Minutes: __________

Water: 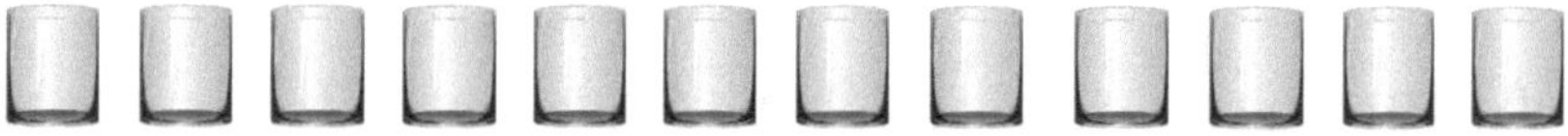

Time	Food Item	Carbs	Carb Balance

How do you feel today?

(Notes)

Date: __________ M Tu W Th F Sa Su

Steps: __________ Exercise Minutes: __________

Water:

Time	Food Item	Carbs	Carb Balance

How do you feel today?

(Notes)

Date: __________ M Tu W Th F Sa Su

clip corner here

Steps: __________ Exercise Minutes: __________

Water:

Time	Food Item	Carbs	Carb Balance

How do you feel today?

(Notes)

Date: __________ M Tu W Th F Sa Su

Steps: __________ Exercise Minutes: __________

Water:

Time	Food Item	Carbs	Carb Balance

How do you feel today?

(Notes)

clip corner here

Date: __________ M Tu W Th F Sa Su

Steps: __________ Exercise Minutes: __________

Water:

Time	Food Item	Carbs	Carb Balance

How do you feel today?

(Notes)

Date: __________ M Tu W Th F Sa Su

Steps: __________ Exercise Minutes: __________

Water:

Time	Food Item	Carbs	Carb Balance

How do you feel today?

(Notes)

Date: __________ M Tu W Th F Sa Su

clip corner here

Steps: __________ Exercise Minutes: __________

Water:

Time	Food Item	Carbs	Carb Balance

How do you feel today?

(Notes)

Date: __________ M Tu W Th F Sa Su

Steps: __________ Exercise Minutes: __________

Water:

Time	Food Item	Carbs	Carb Balance

How do you feel today?

(Notes)

clip corner here

Date: __________ M Tu W Th F Sa Su

Steps: __________ Exercise Minutes: __________

Water:

Time	Food Item	Carbs	Carb Balance

How do you feel today?

(Notes)

Date: __________ M Tu W Th F Sa Su

Steps: __________ Exercise Minutes: __________

Water:

Time	Food Item	Carbs	Carb Balance

How do you feel today?

(Notes)

clip corner here

Date: __________ M Tu W Th F Sa Su

Steps: __________ Exercise Minutes: __________

Water:

Time	Food Item	Carbs	Carb Balance

How do you feel today?

(Notes)

Date: __________ M Tu W Th F Sa Su

Steps: __________ Exercise Minutes: __________

Water:

Time	Food Item	Carbs	Carb Balance

How do you feel today?
(Notes)

Date: __________ M Tu W Th F Sa Su

clip corner here

Steps: __________ Exercise Minutes: __________

Water:

Time	Food Item	Carbs	Carb Balance

How do you feel today?

(Notes)

Date: __________ M Tu W Th F Sa Su

Steps: __________ Exercise Minutes: __________

Water:

Time	Food Item	Carbs	Carb Balance

How do you feel today?

(Notes)

Date: __________ M Tu W Th F Sa Su

clip corner here

Steps: __________ Exercise Minutes: __________

Water:

Time	Food Item	Carbs	Carb Balance

How do you feel today?

(Notes)

Date: __________ M Tu W Th F Sa Su

Steps: __________ Exercise Minutes: __________

Water:

Time	Food Item	Carbs	Carb Balance

How do you feel today?
(Notes)

Date: __________ M Tu W Th F Sa Su

clip corner here

Steps: __________ Exercise Minutes: __________

Water:

Time	Food Item	Carbs	Carb Balance

How do you feel today?

(Notes)

Date: __________ M Tu W Th F Sa Su

Steps: __________ Exercise Minutes: __________

Water:

Time	Food Item	Carbs	Carb Balance

How do you feel today?
(Notes)

clip corner here

Date: __________ M Tu W Th F Sa Su

Steps: __________ Exercise Minutes: __________

Water:

Time	Food Item	Carbs	Carb Balance

How do you feel today?

(Notes)

Date: __________ M Tu W Th F Sa Su

Steps: __________ Exercise Minutes: __________

Water:

Time	Food Item	Carbs	Carb Balance

How do you feel today?
(Notes)

Date: __________ M Tu W Th F Sa Su

clip corner here

Steps: __________ Exercise Minutes: __________

Water:

Time	Food Item	Carbs	Carb Balance

How do you feel today?

(Notes)

Date: __________ M Tu W Th F Sa Su

Steps: __________ Exercise Minutes: __________

Water:

Time	Food Item	Carbs	Carb Balance

How do you feel today?

(Notes)

clip corner here

Date: __________ M Tu W Th F Sa Su

Steps: __________ Exercise Minutes: __________

Water:

Time	Food Item	Carbs	Carb Balance

How do you feel today?

(Notes)

Date: __________ M Tu W Th F Sa Su

Steps: __________ Exercise Minutes: __________

Water:

Time	Food Item	Carbs	Carb Balance

How do you feel today?
(Notes)

clip corner here

Date: __________ M Tu W Th F Sa Su

Steps: __________ Exercise Minutes: __________

Water:

Time	Food Item	Carbs	Carb Balance

How do you feel today?
(Notes)

Date: __________ M Tu W Th F Sa Su

Steps: __________ Exercise Minutes: __________

Water:

Time	Food Item	Carbs	Carb Balance

How do you feel today?
(Notes)

Date: __________ M Tu W Th F Sa Su

clip corner here

Steps: __________ Exercise Minutes: __________

Water: 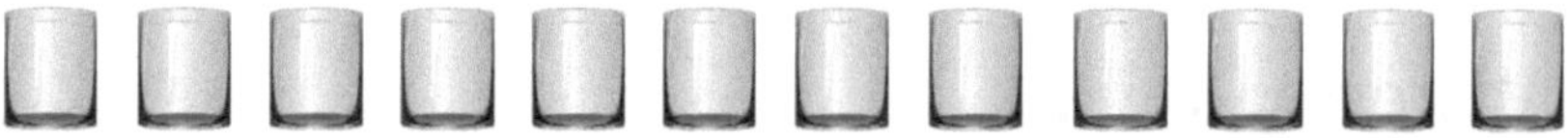

Time	Food Item	Carbs	Carb Balance

How do you feel today?

(Notes)

Date: __________ M Tu W Th F Sa Su

Steps: __________ Exercise Minutes: __________

Water:

Time	Food Item	Carbs	Carb Balance

How do you feel today?

(Notes)

Date: __________ M Tu W Th F Sa Su

clip corner here

Steps: __________ Exercise Minutes: __________

Water:

Time	Food Item	Carbs	Carb Balance

How do you feel today?

(Notes)

Date: ________ M Tu W Th F Sa Su

Steps: ________ Exercise Minutes: ________

Water:

Time	Food Item	Carbs	Carb Balance

How do you feel today?
(Notes)

clip corner here

Date: __________ M Tu W Th F Sa Su

Steps: __________ Exercise Minutes: __________

Water:

Time	Food Item	Carbs	Carb Balance

How do you feel today?

(Notes)

Date: __________ M Tu W Th F Sa Su

Steps: __________ Exercise Minutes: __________

Water:

Time	Food Item	Carbs	Carb Balance

How do you feel today?
(Notes)

Date: __________ M Tu W Th F Sa Su

clip corner here

Steps: __________ Exercise Minutes: __________

Water:

Time	Food Item	Carbs	Carb Balance

How do you feel today?

(Notes)

Date: __________ M Tu W Th F Sa Su

Steps: __________ Exercise Minutes: __________

Water:

Time	Food Item	Carbs	Carb Balance

How do you feel today?

(Notes)

Date: __________ M Tu W Th F Sa Su

clip corner here

Steps: __________ Exercise Minutes: __________

Water:

Time	Food Item	Carbs	Carb Balance

How do you feel today?

(Notes)

Date: __________ M Tu W Th F Sa Su

Steps: __________ Exercise Minutes: __________

Water:

Time	Food Item	Carbs	Carb Balance

How do you feel today?
(Notes)

Date: __________ M Tu W Th F Sa Su

clip corner here

Steps: __________ Exercise Minutes: __________

Water:

Time	Food Item	Carbs	Carb Balance

How do you feel today?

(Notes)

Date: __________ M Tu W Th F Sa Su

Steps: __________ Exercise Minutes: __________

Water:

Time	Food Item	Carbs	Carb Balance

How do you feel today?
(Notes)

clip corner here

Date: __________ M Tu W Th F Sa Su

Steps: __________ Exercise Minutes: __________

Water:

Time	Food Item	Carbs	Carb Balance

How do you feel today?

(Notes)

Date: __________ M Tu W Th F Sa Su

Steps: __________ Exercise Minutes: __________

Water:

Time	Food Item	Carbs	Carb Balance

How do you feel today?

(Notes)

clip corner here

Date: __________ M Tu W Th F Sa Su

Steps: __________ Exercise Minutes: __________

Water:

Time	Food Item	Carbs	Carb Balance

How do you feel today?
(Notes)

Date: __________ M Tu W Th F Sa Su

Steps: __________ Exercise Minutes: __________

Water:

Time	Food Item	Carbs	Carb Balance

How do you feel today?
(Notes)

Date: __________ M Tu W Th F Sa Su

clip corner here

Steps: __________ Exercise Minutes: __________

Water:

Time	Food Item	Carbs	Carb Balance

How do you feel today?
(Notes)

Date: __________ M Tu W Th F Sa Su

Steps: __________ Exercise Minutes: __________

Water:

Time	Food Item	Carbs	Carb Balance

How do you feel today?

(Notes)

Date: __________ M Tu W Th F Sa Su

clip corner here

Steps: __________ Exercise Minutes: __________

Water:

Time	Food Item	Carbs	Carb Balance

How do you feel today?

(Notes)

Date: __________ M Tu W Th F Sa Su

Steps: __________ Exercise Minutes: __________

Water:

Time	Food Item	Carbs	Carb Balance

How do you feel today?
(Notes)

clip corner here

Date: __________ M Tu W Th F Sa Su

Steps: __________ Exercise Minutes: __________

Water:

Time	Food Item	Carbs	Carb Balance

How do you feel today?

(Notes)

Notes / Additional Tracking Information

Notes / Additional Tracking Information

Notes / Additional Tracking Information

Notes / Additional Tracking Information

Also available: How To Journal the Positive Series

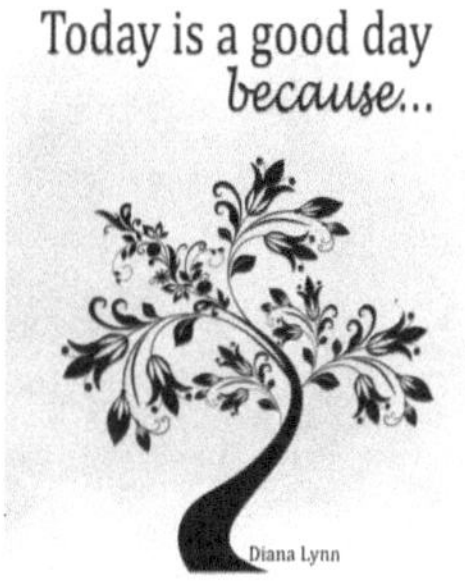

ISBN 978-0-9977516-0-4

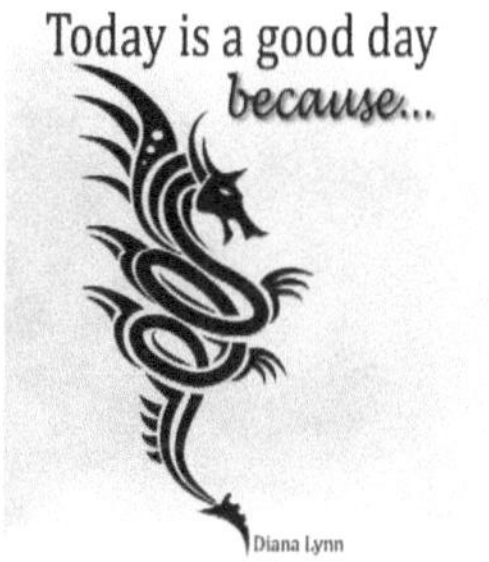

ISBN 978-0-9977516-1-1

D & D Graphics Self-help | Diet | Journaling | Weight Loss

ISBN: 978-0-9982413-2-6
Published by D&D Graphics in 2017
First edition; First printing

website: dianalynnwrites.com

Made in United States
Troutdale, OR
11/03/2026

56844435R00070